Clean Eating: 35 Quick and Easy Healthy Snacks to Help You Burn Fat, Increase Energy and Gain Lean Muscle

Who is this book for?

Do you struggle creating healthy snacks?...

Do you want to eat healthier, but get overwhelmed by having to figure out how to cook healthy?

Most of us want to eat healthier, but we don't know what kind of foods to buy and if we do know what foods to buy, we don't know any tasty recipes we can make with those foods. If this scenario sounds familiar to you than you're someone who needs to read this book.

There are a lot of myths about eating healthy and cooking healthy. One of which being, it's too expensive. Another myth is that it takes too much time. Other things I hear a lot are that it won't taste good or to eat healthy I need to starve myself.

Fortunately for you – none of those myths are true and this book will prove it to you...

You can create healthy snacks for the same amount of money that you can create unhealthy meals. You can create delicious and healthy snacks in 2-15 minutes depending on what you're cooking. The food you will be cooking will not only taste amazing, but it will make you feel amazing. You can eat these snacks every few hours and still lose weight!

Throughout this book I will give you a list of recipes that you can eat everyday that are specifically designed to help you burn fat, increase energy, promote lean muscle growth and make you feel good. The truth is that when you eat healthy meals like the recipes will show you how to do in this book you not only start to look better, but you feel much better as well.

Through my work as a health and performance coach I have had many clients struggle with weight loss and sticking to a healthy lifestyle. One of the biggest things they struggled with was knowing what foods to eat and how to cook healthy snacks with those foods. So many times I had clients asking me what I ate to keep such a sustained healthy lifestyle. I thought I could do everyone in the world, including every past, current and future client the favor of creating this book of recipes on clean eating. There are recipes within this book that will work for everyone. If you cook from this book on a consistent basis, then you will lose weight and feel great. It's as simple as that.

Why these recipes?

Before getting into the first recipe I want to share with you my philosophy on nutrition and why I chose the recipes I did. There are a lot of healthy eating cookbooks out there telling to eat certain ways, but they don't explain why? I believe that the 'Why' is the most important thing to know before adapting a new eating style. Since I am going to tell you what kind of meals to make I believe the least I can do is tell you why!

All the recipes in this book create balanced meals with at least 2 of the 3 macronutrients: Protein, Carbohydrates and Fats. Specifically this book is full of recipes that incorporate lean protein, complex carbohydrates and healthy fats. These 3 types of foods should make up your diet, because they all serve a very specific purpose.

Protein is an essential nutrient that is going to deliver you the amino acids you need to promote healthy muscle and other body tissues. Protein is also a main source of energy for the body. That means we need protein if we want to have healthy muscles and a healthy body.

Carbohydrates are not essential nutrients to the body, but they are amazing place to get energy and micronutrients. That means through carbohydrates the body can get lots of rich calories for energy, as well as nutrients like fiber that promote healthy functioning of the body.

Fats are an essential nutrient for the body that is going to deliver you healthy brain and cell function. Fats are also a main source of energy for the body. That means we need fats to have a healthy brain and a healthy body.

I am not going to go too deep into the benefits of each macronutrient, but the above should give you a brief background on why each one is so important to our overall health. If you would like to see a full list of the healthiest proteins, fats and carbohydrates that we are going to be cooking with you can check out the bonus section at the end of the book where a grocery list is provided for you. If you want to calculate how many calories you are eating each meal you can always check nutritiondata.com to learn more.

Contents Page

Let's get started

This book is split up into four sections where you can quickly flip through and find a recipe that fits your current needs. The four sections are snacks with meat, snacks with no meat, post workout snacks and sweet snacks. These four categories will give you the freedom to choose exactly the type of meal you desire.

The recipes in this book can be considered snacks or small meals. You will see I consistently refer to them as snacks, because my belief is that you should be eating snacks or small meals every three hours. Since you will be eating so frequently none of these meals are exceptionally heavy. That's why they can be referred to as healthy and balanced snacks. If you're ready to dive into this recipe book and start cooking and eating healthier than ever then **let's get started...**

Section 1: Snacks with Meat

Recipe #1: The Bold Burrito Bowl

Black Beans – 1/2 cup

Free Range Chicken – 3 ounces

Avocado - whole large avocado

Salsa – 2 tbsp

Chopped Onions – ¼ cup

Fresh Cracked Black Pepper – 1 tsp

Stats:

Protein – 28 grams

Fat – 30 grams

Carbs – 20 grams

Total Calories – 462 calories

Serving Size: Serves 1

Instructions: *Cook chicken and black beans separately. Chop vegetables. Put all of the ingredients together in a bowl and add as much salsa as you desire.*

Recipe #2: Taco Salad

Romaine lettuce or spinach – 4 cups

Purple Cabbage – ¼ cup

Salsa – 2 tbsp

Free Range Chicken – 3 ounces

Black Beans – 1/2 cup

Avocado – whole large avocado

Chopped Tomatoes – ¼ cup

Chopped Onions – ¼ cup

Cilantro – 2 tbsp

Stats:

Protein – 28 grams

Fat – 30 grams

Carbs – 20 grams

Total Calories – 462 calories

Serving Size: Serves 1

Instructions: *Cook chicken and black beans separately. Chop vegetables. Put all of the ingredients together in a bowl and add as much salsa as you desire.*

Recipe #3: Quinoa Salmon Bowl

Quinoa – 1 cup

Salmon – 3 ounces

Avocado – whole large avocado

Diced Cucumber – ¼ cucumber

Stats:

Protein – 26 grams

Fat – 30 grams

Carbs – 20 grams

Total Calories – 454 calories

Serving Size: Serves 1

Instructions: *Cook Salmon and Quinoa separately. Chop vegetables. Put all of the ingredients together in on a plate and serve.*

Recipe #4: Tuna Salad

Spinach – 4 cups

Olive Oil – 2 tbsp

Cucumber – 1/3 cucumber

Balsamic Vinegar – 1 tbsp

Tuna – 1 can

Vegan Mayo – 2 tbsp

Black Pepper – 1 tsp

Lemon – 1 tsp

Avocado –whole large avocado

Stats:

Protein – 42 grams

Fat – 46 grams

Carbs – 6 grams

Total Calories – 606 calories

Serving Size: Serves 1

Instructions: *Mix tuna, mayo and pepper. Chop vegetables. Add tuna to vegetables and drizzle lemon juice, olive oil and vinegar on top the salad.*

Recipe #5: Curry Chicken

Free Range Chicken – 3 ounces

Brown Rice – ½ cup

Red Peppers – ¼ cup

White Onions – ¼ cup

Cumin – 2 tsp

Garlic powder – 2 tsp

Coconut Oil – 2 tbsp

Stats:

Protein – 26 grams

Fat – 28 grams

Carbs – 25 grams

Total Calories – 456 calories

Serving Size: Serves 1

Instructions: *Cook chicken and brown rice separately. Grill peppers and onions in coconut oil. Add all ingredients together and add seasoning.*

Recipe #6: Tuna Wrap

Tuna – 1 can

Brown Rice Wrap – 1 wrap

Vegan Mayo – 2 tbsp

Black pepper – 1 tsp

Sriracha – 1 tsp

Avocado – whole large avocado

Chopped onions – ¼ cup

Stats:

Protein – 50 grams

Fat – 26 grams

Carbs – 40 grams

Total Calories – 594 calories

Serving Size: Serves 1

Instructions: *Mix tuna, mayo and pepper together. Warm brown rice wrap in a pan. Add vegetables and tuna to wrap and drizzle sriracha.*

Recipe #7: BBQ Chicken Wrap

Free Range Chicken – 3 ounces

Avocado- whole large avocado

Brown Rice Wrap – 1 wrap

Chopped Tomatoes – 1/4 cup

Romaine Lettuce – 1 cup

BBQ sauce – 1 tbsp

Stats:

Protein – 31 grams

Fat – 22 grams

Carbs – 40 grams

Total Calories – 482 calories

Serving Size: Serves 1

Instructions: *Cook chicken. Warm brown rice wrap in a pan. Add vegetables and chicken to wrap and drizzle BBQ sauce.*

Recipe #8: Omelet with The Works

Eggs – 3 eggs

Mushrooms – ¼ cup

Onions – ¼ cup

Red Peppers – ¼ cup

Sausage – 1 ounce

Ham – 1 ounce

Black Pepper – 1 tsp

Avocado – whole large avocado

Your choice of hot sauce – 1 tsp

Stats:

Protein – 32 grams

Fat – 39 grams

Carbs – 5 grams

Total Calories – 499 calories

Serving Size: Serves 1

Instructions: *Mix eggs, meat and vegetables together and cook to perfection. Place avocado, pepper and hot sauce on top the omelet.*

Recipe #9: Egg Salad Wrap

Eggs – 3 eggs

Brown Rice Wrap – 1 wrap

Vegan Mayo – 1 tbsp

Mustard – 2 tsp

Cayenne Powder – 1 tsp

Black Pepper – 1 tsp

Avocado – whole large avocado

Stats:

Protein – 28 grams

Fat – 28 grams

Carbs – 40 grams

Total Calories – 524 calories

Serving Size: Serves 1

Instructions: *Cook 3 hard boiled eggs. Mix in hard boiled eggs with mayo, mustard, cayenne and pepper. Warm brown rice wrap. Add eggs and avocado to wrap.*

Recipe #10: Teriyaki Beef Bowl

Grass Fed Beef – 3 ounces

Brown Rice – ½ cup

Red and Green Peppers – ¼ cup

Mushrooms – ¼ cup

White Onions – ¼ cup

Sesame Seeds – 2 tbsp

Teriyaki Sauce – 2 tsp

Coconut Oil – 2 tbsp

Stats:

Protein – 30 grams

Fat – 36 grams

Carbs – 22 grams

Total Calories – 532 calories

Serving Size: Serves 1

Instructions: *Cook beef, brown rice and vegetables separately in coconut oil. Mix together when fully cooked and add sesame seeds and teriyaki sauce on top.*

Recipe #11: Steak Stir Fry

Grass Fed Steak – 3 ounces

Red and Green Peppers – ¼ cup

Mushrooms – ¼ cup

White Onions – ¼ cup

Sweet Potatoes – 1/2 cup

Coconut Oil – 2 tbsp

Stats:

Protein – 23 grams

Fat – 28 grams

Carbs – 21 grams

Total Calories – 428 calories

Serving Size: Serves 1

Instructions: *Grill steak and vegetables separately in coconut oil. Add together when cooked and enjoy.*

Recipe #12: Beef Jerky and Almonds

Beef Jerky – 3 ounces

Almonds – 1/2 cup

Stats:

Protein – 36 grams

Fat – 36 grams

Carbs – 11 grams

Total Calories – 512 calories

Serving Size: Serves 1

Instructions: *Eat jerky and almonds separately.*

Recipe #13: Shrimp Salad

Shrimp – 3 ounces

Quinoa – 1 cup

Spinach – 2 cups

Olive Oil – 2 tbsp

Lemon – 1 tsp

Fresh Cracked Black Pepper – 1 tsp

Stats:

Protein – 26 grams

Fat – 35 grams

Carbs – 20 grams

Total Calories – 499 calories

Serving Size: Serves 1

Instructions: *Cook shrimp and quinoa separately. Add both on top of spinach salad. Drizzle lemon, olive oil and pepper on top.*

Section 2: Snacks with No Meat

Recipe #14: The Veggie Vurrito Bowl

Black Beans – 1 cup

Avocado – whole large avocado

Salsa – 3 tbsp

Stats:

Protein – 15 grams

Fat – 29 grams

Carbs – 45 grams

Total Calories – 501 calories

Serving Size: Serves 1

Instructions: *Cook black beans. Mix in sliced avocado and salsa.*

Recipe #15: Almonds, Carrots and Hummus

Almonds – 1/2 cup

Carrots – 1 cup

Hummus – 4 tbsp

Stats:

Protein – 16 grams

Fat – 40 grams

Carbs – 24 grams

Total Calories – 520 calories

Serving Size: Serves 1

Instructions: *Eat almonds separate. Dip carrots into the hummus.*

Recipe #16: Walnuts and Celery

Walnuts – 1/2 cup

Celery sticks – 4 sticks

Hummus – 4 tbsp

Stats:

Protein – 16 grams

Fat – 40 grams

Carbs – 4 grams

Total Calories – 440 calories

Serving Size: Serves 1

Instructions: *Eat walnuts separate. Dip celery sticks into the hummus.*

Recipe #17: Hemp seeds, Broccoli and Hummus

Hemp seeds – 6 tbsp

Broccoli – ½ cup

Hummus – 4 tbsp

Stats:

Protein – 22 grams

Fat – 28 grams

Carbs – 8 grams

Total Calories – 372 calories

Serving Size: Serves 1

Instructions: *Eat hemp seeds separate. Dip broccoli into the hummus.*

Recipe #18: Almond Power Shake

Chocolate Vegan Protein Powder – 1 scoop

Cacao 1 tbsp

Almond butter – 2 tbsp

Oats – 1/2 cup

Ice – ½ cup

Water – ½ cup

Stats:

Protein – 45 grams

Fat – 42 grams

Carbs – 27 grams

Total Calories – 666 calories

Serving Size: Serves 1

Instructions: *Add all ingredients and blend to perfection.*

Recipe #19: Cashew Power Shake

Water – ½ cup

Ice – ½ cup

Cacao 1 tbsp

Cashew Butter 2 tbsp

Chocolate Vegan Protein Powder – 1 scoop

Unsweetened Vanilla Hemp Milk – ¼ cup

Stats:

Protein – 41 grams

Fat – 39 grams

Carbs – 16 grams

Total Calories – 579 calories

Serving Size: Serves 1

Instructions: *Add all ingredients and blend to perfection.*

Recipe #20: Coconut Power Shake

Unsweetened Vanilla Coconut Milk – ½ cup

Water ¼ Cup

Ice – ½ cup

Coconut Peanut Butter 2 tbsp

Vanilla Vegan Protein Powder – 1 scoop

Blend

Stats:

Protein – 39 grams

Fat – 34 grams

Carbs – 6 grams

Total Calories – 486 calories

Serving Size: Serves 1

Instructions: *Add all ingredients and blend to perfection.*

Recipe #21: The Green Machine

Water – ½ cup

Ice - ½ cup

Coconut Oil - 2 tbsp

Chocolate Vegan Protein Powder – 1 scoop

Spinach - 1 cup

Cucumber – ¼ cucumber

Stats:

Protein – 24 grams

Fat – 30 grams

Carbs – 0 grams

Total Calories – 366 calories

Serving Size: Serves 1

Instructions: *Add all ingredients and blend to perfection.*

Recipe #22: Garbanzo Bean Salad

Spinach – 4 cups

Cucumber – ¼ cucumber

Tomato – ½ tomato

Garbanzo Beans – 1 cup

Olive Oil – 2 tbsp

Balsamic Vinegar – 1 tbsp

Alfalfa Sprouts – ¼ cup

Stats:

Protein – 16 grams

Fat – 35 gram

Carbs – 43 grams

Total Calories – 551 calories

Serving Size: Serves 1

Instructions: *Prepare salad; add cold garbanzo beans, olive oil and vinegar on top.*

Recipe #23: Split Pea Mash

Split peas – 1 cup

Fresh Cracked Black Pepper – 1 tsp

Stats:

Protein – 16 grams

Fat – 1 gram

Carbs – 24 grams

Total Calories – 169 calories

Serving Size: Serves 1

Instructions: *Cook split peas and serve with black pepper on top.*

Recipe #24: Asian Salad

Broccoli Slaw – ½ cup

Spinach – 1 cup

Walnuts – ¼ cup

Sesame Oil – 1 tbsp

Tofu – 3 oz

Sriracha – 1 tsp

Stats:

Protein – 20 grams

Fat – 48 grams

Carbs – 2 grams

Total Calories – 520 grams

Serving Size: Serves 1

Instructions: *Cook tofu in a pan. Add to salad, drizzle sesame oil and walnuts on top.*

Recipe #25: Spinach and Hemp Seed Salad

Spinach – 4 cups

Hemp seeds – 3 tbsp

Olive Oil – 2 tbsp

Balsamic Vinegar – 1 tbsp

Stats:

Protein – 14 grams

Fat – 45 grams

Carbs – 3 grams

Total Calories – 473 calories

Serving Size: Serves 1

Instructions: *Prepare salad and then drizzle olive oil, vinegar and hemp seeds on top.*

Section 3: Post Workout Meals

Recipe #26: Vanilla Strawberry Banana Swirl

Veggie Vanilla Protein Powder – 2 scoops

Frozen Strawberries – 1/2 cup

Frozen bananas – 1/2 cup

Ice

Water – 1 cup

Stats:

Protein – 48 grams

Fat – 0 grams

Carbs – 20 grams

Total Calories – 272 calories

Serving Size: Serves 1

Instructions: *Add all ingredients and blend to perfection.*

Recipe #27: Chocolate Blueberry Delight

Veggie Chocolate Protein Powder – 2 scoops

Frozen Blueberries – 1 cup

Water – 1 cup

Stats:

Protein – 48 grams

Fat – 0 grams

Carbs – 20 grams

Total Calories – 272 calories

Serving Size: Serves 1

Instructions: *Add all ingredients and blend to perfection.*

Recipe #28: Bar and Pineapple

Protein bar of choice (Quest or Think Thin)

Pineapple 1 cup

Stats:

Protein – 20 grams

Fat – 6 grams

Carbs – 27 grams

Total Calories – 242 calories

Serving Size: Serves 1

Instructions: *Add all ingredients and blend to perfection.*

Recipe #29: Choco-Berry

Chocolate Whey Protein Powder – 2 scoops

Frozen Mixed Berries 1 cup

Water – 1 cup

Stats:

Protein – 50 grams

Fat – 0 grams

Carbs – 18 grams

Total Calories – 272 calories

Serving Size: Serves 1

Instructions: *Add all ingredients and blend to perfection.*

Recipe #30: Sweet Vanilla

Vanilla Whey Protein Powder – 2 scoops

Dextrose – 2 tbsp

Water – 1 cup

Stats:

Protein – 50 grams

Fat – 0 grams

Carbs – 20 grams

Total Calories – 280 calories

Serving Size: Serves 1

Instructions: *Add all ingredients and blend to perfection.*

Section 4: Healthy Sweets

Recipe #31: Apple and Almond Butter

Green Apple – 1 whole

Natural Almond Butter – 2 tbsp

Stats:

Protein – 14 grams

Fat – 34 grams

Carbs – 21 grams

Total Calories – 446 calories

Serving Size: Serves 1

Instructions: *Slice apple and spread almond butter on each piece.*

Recipe #32: Apple and Peanut Butter

Green Apple – 1 whole

Natural Peanut Butter – 2 tbsp

Stats:

Protein – 14 grams

Fat – 34 grams

Carbs – 17 grams

Total Calories – 430 calories

Serving Size: Serves 1

Instructions: *Slice apple and spread peanut butter on each piece.*

Recipe #33: Apple and Cashew Butter

Green Apple – 1 whole

Natural Cashew Butter – 2 tbsp

Stats:

Protein – 8 grams

Fat – 34 grams

Carbs – 30 grams

Total Calories – 458 calories

Serving Size: Serves 1

Instructions: *Slice apple and spread cashew butter on each piece.*

Recipe #34: Hemp Milkshake

Unsweetened Vanilla Hemp Milk – ½ cup

Cacao – 2 tbsp

Vanilla Vegan Protein Powder – 1 scoop

Ice – ½ cup

Natural Almond Butter – 2 tbsp

Stats:

Protein – 52 grams

Fat – 48 grams

Carbs – 6 grams

Total Calories – 664 calories

Serving Size: Serves 1

Instructions: *Add all ingredients and blend to perfection.*

Recipe #35: Coconut Milkshake

Unsweetened Vanilla Coconut Milk – ½ cup

Cacao – 2 tbsp

Chocolate Espresso Vegan Protein Powder – 1 scoop

Ice – ½ cup

Natural Almond Butter – 2 tbsp

Stats:

Protein – 52 grams

Fat – 48 grams

Carbs – 6 grams

Total Calories – 664 calories

Serving Size: Serves 1

Instructions: *Add all ingredients and blend to perfection.*

Bonus Content: Grocery List

Below is a grocery list that will help you pick out all the foods necessary to eat clean while cooking all the recipes in this book.

Complex Carb List	Healthy Fat List	Healthy Proteins
Yams/Sweet Potatoes	Avocados	Plant Based Protein Powder
Black Beans	Olive Oil	Whey Protein Powder
Brown Rice	Coconut Oil	Tempeh
Quinoa	Krill Oil	Tofu
Oatmeal	Flax Seeds	Eggs (cage free)
Apples	Walnuts	Chicken (free range)
Brown Rice Wraps	Almonds	Beef (grass fed)
Garbanzo Beans	Natural Nut Butters	*High protein
beans/nuts	ex: peanut/almond	Fish
Split Peas	Pine Nuts	Shelled Seafood
Vegetables (See Glossary)	Sunflower Seeds	
Low Carb Wraps	Chia Seeds	
	Hemp Seeds	
	Pistachios	
	Vegan Cheese	
	Cacao	
	Pumpkin Seeds	
	Brazil Nuts	

Vegetable list

- Asparagus
- Broccoli
- Spinach
- Celery
- Cucumber
- Lettuce
- Sprouts
- Wheatgrass
- Parsley
- Cilantro
- Misc. Fresh Herbs
- Brussel Sprouts
- Bok Choy
- Kale
- Artichoke
- Bell Peppers (all kinds)
- Bean Sprouts
- Cabbage (all kinds)
- Edamame
- Garlic
- Ginger

- Beets
- Swiss Chard
- Mushrooms
- Peas (all kinds)
- Squash
- Zucchini
- Water Chestnuts
- Radishes
- Lemon (fruit exception)
- Lime (fruit exception)
- Tomato (fruit exception)
- Onion (fruit exception)
- Green beans

Another Super Helpful Kindle Book!

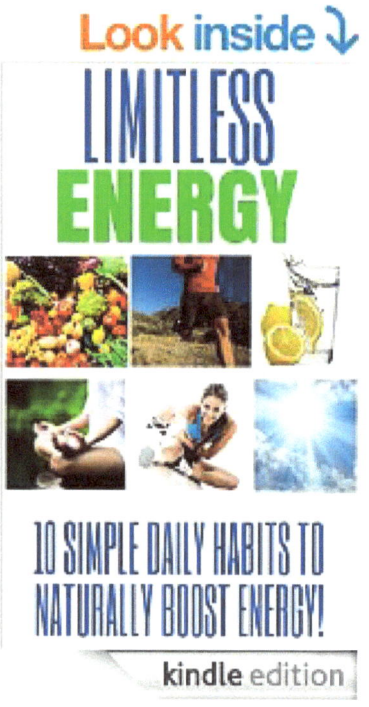

Limitless Energy:

Mastering your nutrition is a massive first step towards creating abundant energy in your everyday life. If you want to take your energy to a whole new level then check out my other book.

Do you want more Energy?

Do you often feel tired and run down throughout your day and wish you could just magically flip a switch and feel energized?

Most of us try to flip this switch by consuming cup after cup of coffee or other caffeinated products, simply so that we can feel normal. If this scenario sounds familiar to you than you're someone who needs to read this book.

If you have tried everything from caffeine to vitamins, to energy shots, to nicotine to Adderall and everything in between without achieving the results you desired – then you are in the vast majority. Most people yo-yo their energy up and down with stimulants that are helpful for a short time, but ultimately lead to a crash and/or other negative health side effects. Not to mention that over time they can become really expensive.

Fortunately for you - there's another option...

You CAN have lasting energy and motivation without the crash and you can do it all naturally. The contents in this book will walk you step by step through the top ten best habits and natural techniques for improving energy, motivation and overall happiness and health.

Check out my #1 best selling health/fitness kindle book to learn the habits to creating limitless energy

Final Words

My intention for this book was to give you an incredibly valuable resource that you can use to empower yourself to living a healthier and happier life. Sometimes life happens and we're not able to eat quite as healthy as we would like to, but with this book as your guide you make a deliberate choice to eat healthy whenever you have access to the foods on your grocery list (see bonus section).

Every meal is an opportunity for you to start a new eating habit. Remember that your past doesn't equal your future. All it takes is one healthy meal to set you back on the right path towards living a healthy lifestyle. Ideally you will be using this recipe book to craft all of your meals and create a sustainable nutrition program that fits into your new lifestyle. Remember this is NOT a diet recipe. This is a nutritional resource to help you eat healthier meals for the rest of your life.

Think of the recipe book this way. The more recipes you make using this book or the more you eat from the grocery list attached – the better you will look and feel. The foods on the grocery list are largely comprised of super foods that help you burn fat, gain energy, gain lean muscle, promote healthy cell function and boost your immune system. You now have the knowledge you need create the meals that are going to make you healthier and happier, so get to cookin!

Quick note. If you enjoyed this book, pleaseeee take 30 seconds to share your positive thoughts and post them as a review on my Amazon Book page! Your review means so much to me and it helps spread the word about how we can all be cooking healthy and delicious meals every day.

Finally, I want to commend you for making it through this book. Your commitment to getting better is truly inspirational. You will be rewarded for your efforts with a body that looks and feels better than ever if you continue to cook using the recipes and foods in this book.

If you have any questions about concepts in this book you can email me at..

Brandon@EntrepreneurFitness.com

or if you want to learn more about living a healthy lifestyle you can check out my site at http://www.entrepreneurfitness.com.

There you can join my email list to connect, learn more strategies and gain inspiration for improving your physical, mental and emotional well-being.

www.ingramcontent.com/pod-product-compliance
Lightning Source LLC
Chambersburg PA
CBHW060838290526
45792CB00006BB/1973